Essential Oils for Kids:

4 DIY Natural Toxic-Free Recipes For Your Children's Health

Table of content:

Introduction

You're looking for a better way to care for your kids...

You take them to the doctor, give them the best of meals, and make sure nothing happens to them within your power. The problem is you're getting disillusioned with prescription drugs, additives in food, and other chemicals in what they drink, you are looking for a better way to maintain their health to reduce the number of times you have to take them to the doctor for health or other problems.

You've looked online and even talked to a few people who sell essential oils, but all the information is either too much to digest or it seems to contradict itself. Look no further, this book was written with 20+ years experience in the natural health and aromatherapy fields. I will give you all the advice you need to get started with essential oils, and aromatherapy, and helping you to raise your children in a toxic-free environment.

Chapter 1 - Aromatherapy for Kids 101

There are over 90 essential oils on the market, and all of them are used for all sorts of health benefits, but not all are appropriate for children. Different age groups can only use certain essential oils. Out of the over 90 essential oils, there are less than 30 essential oils that are safe for use for children.

Aromatherapy Preparations

From simple blends to soaps and shampoos, there are a lot of ways you can prepare essential oils. Here is a list of them you can do at home:

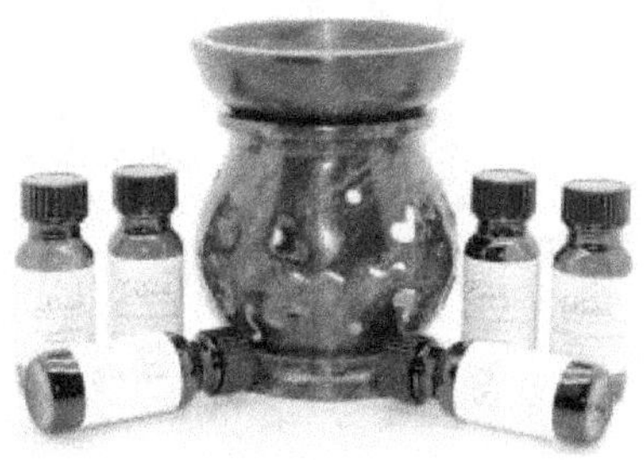

1. Simple Diffuser Blend

This is mixing different essential oils together and placing the mixture either in a diffuser or on a candle warmer.

2. Bath/Mineral Salts

This is a combination of epsom and sea salts with borax and baking soda or ground oatmeal with essential oils and carrier oils. You add it to a bath for different health reasons.

3. Shampoo

You add either add essential oils to an existing shampoo or make your own shampoo from home and control what goes into your shampoo.

4. Soaps

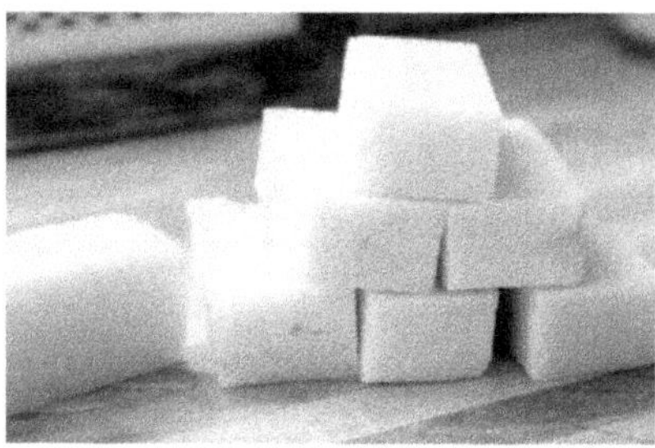

There are melt and pour soaps you can make yourself and add essential oils to.

5. Room Sprays

These are very simply essential blends that have been added to water in a spray bottle to freshen a room or sanitize an area.

6. Massage Oils

These oils can be used as chest rubs and other things for children.

7. Salves and ointments

These are aromatherapy products made from petroleum jelly or bees wax. It will help to keep the essential oils on the area you are trying to treat longer.

Like most hobbies, you need the proper tools to do a proper job, and aromatherapy is no different. Here is a list of tools you will need to make the preparations, and most are already in your kitchen.

Glass Double Boiler

This will come in handy when making salves and ointments. You can also make your own double boiler by placing a glass bowl in a small pot that has boiling water.

Crock Pot

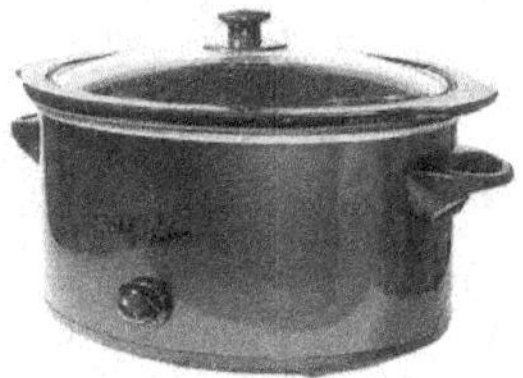

When your making melt and pour soap, you need something to melt in that is bigger than a double boiler. That's where a crock pot comes into play.

Soap Molds

You can find these in any craft shop as well as online. They range from loaf shapes to more artistic molds so you can be creative.

Empty Shampoo Bottles

These can be bottles that you have emptied and cleaned. This will save you a little bit of money.

Air-Tight Containers

They come in all shapes and sizes and you can find them online. They will be a life-saver when making salves and ointments. You can also use them to store your bath and mineral salts.

Measuring cups/spoons

These will help you measure out all the ingredients you will need to make the preparations.

Food Scale

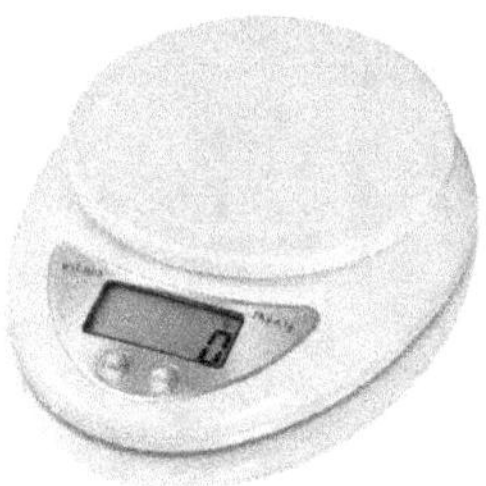

This is for weighing and measuring your dry ingredients like the baking soda and blocks of melt and pour soap.

Spray Bottles

These are for mixing the sanitizing sprays and room sprays.

Wooden Spoons

These are recommend to mix the ingredients when making soaps, ointments, and salves. You can even use silicone mixing tools, if you like.

Blender/Food Processor

This is to mix the shampoos, dry goods and other ingredients together.

Gloves

You need to use these to mix the essential oils. Essential oils can cause contact dermatitis when used undiluted.

Baking Soda

This is a common ingredient in bath salts and mineral baths.

Borax

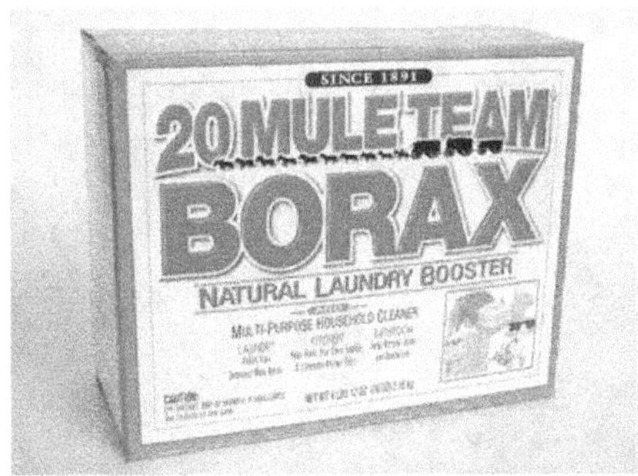

This is a naturally occurring mineral that helps to smooth the skin.

Epsom Salts

This is one of the two salts used in a mineral or bath salts.

Ground Oatmeal

This is usually steel cut oats that have been ground into a fine powder for use in baths. It's used in place of salts in cases of high blood pressure.

Melt and Pour Soap

This can be found in any craft shop or online. It comes in bricks that are graded so you can cut them in ounce increments.

Carrier Oils

These are oils you add essential oils to in order to dilute them.

Labels

It's always good to label your products and date them. Many preparations lose their punch after a certain amount of time and others have to be used immediately.

Salves have a shelf life of 6 months.

Ointments have a shelf life of up to a year.

Shampoos have a shelf life of four months.

Melt and Pour Soaps have a shelf life of up to a year.

There are a few things you need to keep in mind when using essential oils:

1. Store in a cool dry place

Essential oils have a habit of evaporating in high temperatures. To avoid this, store your essential oils in a cool dry place, like a pantry.

2. Keep undiluted essential oils out of little ones' reach

Essential oils are toxic undiluted and can cause health issues.

3. Clean your tools before and after use.

This will prevent cross-contamination. You can buy tools just for making the preparations, but since you're not dealing with really caustic materials, it isn't really necessary.

4. Do not ingest essential oils

Some would say this is perfectly safe to do, and I would say only in small doses and mixed into food. It does not matter the grade of essential oil. If it is not diluted, it should not be ingested.

5. Patch Test

This the practice of diluting a small amount of an essential oil and placing it on a small patch of skin to see if you have an adverse reaction to it. This should be performed for all essential oils you are planning on using.

2 drops of essential oil

1 tsp vegetable oil

Mix together and apply a small amount to a patch of skin that is not readily visible. If no reaction is seen within 24 hours, the essential oil is safe to use.

6. Do not use undiluted essential oils on the skin.

Some companies would have you believe this is perfectly fine if they are therapeutic grade essential oils. This is simply not true. Even Lavender, an essential oil commonly used undiluted, can cause contact dermatitis when used too often undiluted.

7. Do not put on infant hands and feet

There are sites out there that say this is a good idea due to the nerves in the hands and feet, and it is, but babies have a tendency of putting their feet and hands in their mouths. So, it's best not to do it.

8. Know where your essential oil is coming from.

Vet the manufacturer and look at how they are rated in terms of purity and how the screen their essential oils. There are companies out there that will try to substitute one essential for another or dilute the oil and not advertise it is diluted.

As you can see, I'm already debunking some information that is out there. Now, let's get on to the rest of the book, starting with the immune system.

Chapter 2 - Essential Oil List

As I mentioned in the previous chapter, not all essential oils are suitable for children under twelve. Here is a list of essential oils and the age groups most appropriate for them. Starting with newborn, you can add the essential oils to the list for the other age groups, but you can not add them in regression.

For instance you can add the newborn essential oils to the 2-12 month list, but you cannot add the 2-12 month list to the newborn essential oil list.

Newborn *Dill (Anethum graveolens)*

This essential oil is good for colic, flatulence, and indigestion

Lavender (Lavandula angustufolia)

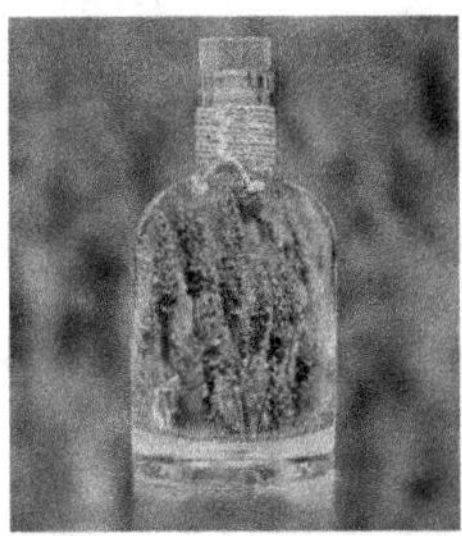

Lavender is the most versatile of the essential oils. You can combine it with virtually every other oil in the market; you can use undiluted sparingly without side effects, and it can be used for a multitude of health reasons:

Dermatitis, earache, eczema, psoriasis, sunburn muscle aches, asthma, bronchitis, whooping cough, colic, flatulence, nausea, flu, insomnia, headache, nervous tension, and dry scalp. That is just the short list.

Roman Chamomile (*Chamaemelum nobile*)

Highly recommended for sensitive skin, this essential oil has a long list of benefits as well:

Acne, allergies, dermatitis, earache, eczema, insect bites, rashes, nausea, indigestion, colic, insomnia, and nervous tension to name a few.

Yarrow (*Achillea millefolium*)

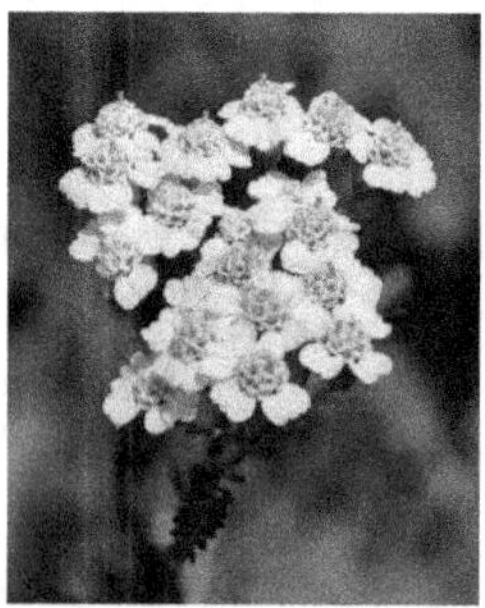

This essential oil is not as famous as the two above it, but it does come in handy for helping with acne, the treatment of burns, eczema, rashes, lessening scars, toning the skin, cramps, flatulence, indigestion, colds, breaking fevers, flu, insomnia, an is often added to hair rinses.

2-12 Months

Geranium (*Pelargonium graveolens*)

This floral oil has been used in the treatment of bruises, burns, congested skin, dermatitis, eczema, oily complexions, tonsillitis, sore throats, and nervous tension. *Can cause dermatitis in highly sensitive skin.*

Tangerine/Mandarin (Citrus reticulata)

This essential oil is labeled as one or the other in most natural health stores and online. This is why I include the Latin name of the oil. This oil is known to help with congested and oily skin, lightening of scars, a skin toner, intestinal problems, digestive problems, insomnia, nervous tension, and restlessness.

Eucalyptus (Eucalyptus globulus)

Well known for being used in vaporizers and other diffusion devices, eucalyptus has been used to open nasal passages and congested chests. It can also help treat insect bites, skin infections, ease muscular aches and pains, sprains, and throat infections. It is also effective in treating bronchitis, sinusitis, colds, flu, and measles.

Tea Tree (Melaleuca alternifolia)

This essential oil is the perfect substitute for use in killing mold, mildew and bacteria. It is also used to treat acne, athlete's foot, burns, cold sores, dandruff, insect bites, oily skin, rashes, asthma, bronchitis, coughs, sinusitis, whooping cough, thrush, colds, fever, flu, chicken pox, measles.

12 Months-5 Years

Palmarosa (Cymnopogon martinii)

This essential oil has been known to help with acne, dermatitis, minor skin infections, scarring, facials, oily skin, dry skin, intestinal infections.

5 Years - 12 Years

Clary Sage (Salvia sclarea)

This is another strong essential oil, but it's good for use in this age rage. Since it is a little more potent than the ones before it, I would not recommend making it the mainstay of a blend. Two to three drops should be enough for a tablespoon. This oil is good to help with acne, dandruff, oily skin and hair, muscular aches and pains, intestinal cramps and flatulence.

Nutmeg (Myristica fragrans)

This aromatic oil is used for helping treat muscular aches and pains, flatulence, indigestion, nausea, and bacterial infections. *This essential oil is toxic in large doses.*

Chapter 3 - The Immune System

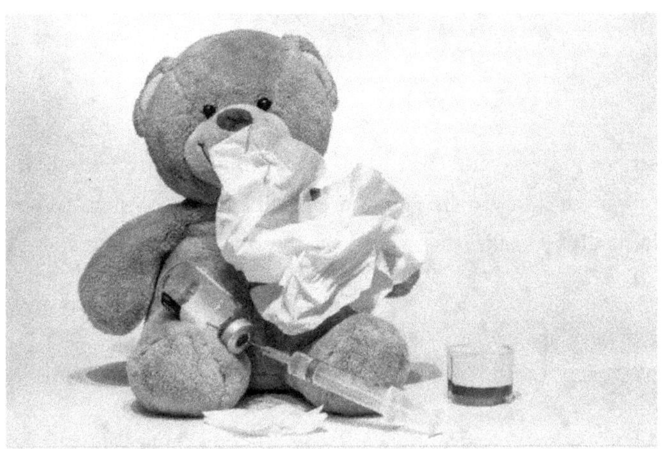

This is the system that fights infections, colds, the flu and other diseases. In today's world it's unheard of to let our children play outside barefoot, drink out of water hoses, and even just get muddy for fear of germs, but did you know depriving them of that actually isn't good for their immune system? Your body is constantly exposed to a germ-filled environment on a daily basis. This allows your immune system to adapt to the bombardment and become stronger. This is the same for your children. We want to provide a sterile environment for them, but that does not allow their immune systems to become as strong as they need to be to cope with everyday bacteria and germs.

There are some things you can do to help their immune system prevent them from getting sick:

1. They need plenty of sleep

Toddlers 1-3 years: 11-14 hours of sleep
Preschoolers 3-5 years: 10-13 hours of sleep
6-13 years: 9-11 hours

This may seem like a lot, but they are still developing their immune systems, and they need all the rest they can get. This is why it is recommended toddlers to 5 years of age need to take naps.

2. Balanced diet

Fruits, vegetables, meats, grains, fats, and the rest of the pyramid in a proper balance is essential to the development of a growing child and their immune system. When you start them early on healthy snacks, they will carry that habit with them as they grow.

3. Let them play

Between day care or school, chores, and homework, there is one thing that can get lost in the shuffle at times, play. They need to go outside and play, whether it be on a bicycle or in-line skates, playing a sport, or just pretending they're Jedi or superheroes, children need to play. It's good their immune system and their imagination.

4. Spending time with them

Your children need you to spend quality time with them. This time can mean watching shows with them, playing catch, or even reading them a bedtime story. They need their parents to interact with them to form bonds, and be reassured they are loved. It's one thing to a child to be told they are loved. It's Quite another when you show it to them.

Chest Rub

When your child's chest is congested, you want to do anything you can to alleviate the coughing and hacking. Here are a couple of recipes you can use to help them breathe and sleep better. It will also boost the

Newborn Chest Rub

1/2 Cup Coconut oil

1 tbsp beeswax pastilles (Little beads)

2 tbsp Shea butter

5 Drops Lavender essential oil

5 Drops Yarrow Essential oil

- In a double boiler, place the coconut oil, beeswax, and Shea Butter.
- Mix the essential oils and set aside
- Stir until it is melted.
- Place in a tightly lidded container.
- When it is still warm and not hot, stir in the essential oils
- To use, spread a light layer on the chest.

12 Months to 5 Years Chest Rub

1/2 Cup Coconut oil

1 tbsp beeswax pastilles (Little beads)

2 tbsp Shea butter

5 Drops Eucalyptus Essential oil

5 Drops Mandarin Essential oil

5 Drops Geranium Essential oil

- In a double boiler, place the coconut oil, beeswax, and Shea Butter.
- Mix the essential oils and set aside
- Stir until it is melted.
- Place in a tightly lidded container.
- When it is still warm and not hot, stir in the essential oils
- To use, spread a light layer on the chest.

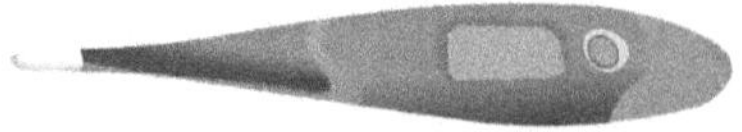

Nothing stops us in our tracks faster than kissing our child on the forehead and feeling it is hot to the touch. Our first instinct is always to call the doctor and then reach for something to break the fever. A fever is the immune system's way of fighting off the infection by burning it out of the system. I am not saying to let the fever rage. I saying it is better to regulate the fever instead of trying to keep it down until it breaks. This will give the body a fighting chance to get rid of the infection that is inside the body trying to take hold.

There is one circumstance in which you need to need to go to the emergency room when your child has a fever:

When the fever is in a steady increase no matter what you have done to regulate it, and it's been constantly rising for the course of the day.

Here are the limits of the temperatures of your child and when you need to take them to the doctor:

3-6 mos. 101F
Over 6 mos: 103F+
Any age: 104F+

You can control the temperature of the child by placing them in a bath that matches their body temperature at the time and then slowly introducing cool water to lower the water temperature.

Do not place a child with a fever in an ice bath.

Their system will go into shock because of the extreme temperature change.

2-12 Month Fever Bath

1 Cup Epsom Salts

1/4 Cup Sea Salt

1/4 Cup Baking Soda

5 drops Yarrow Essential Oil

5 Drops Tea Tree Essential Oil

3 Tbsp Sweet Almond Oil

- Mix the dry ingredients and set aside
- Mix the oils together and add to the dry ingredients
- Place in container with a tight lid overnight
- Place an 1/8 cup of the salts in running water and mix well.

12 Months -5 Years Fever Bath

1 Cup Epsom Salts

1/4 Cup Sea Salt

1/4 Cup Baking Soda

5 drops Eucalyptus Essential Oil

5 Drops Tea Tree Essential Oil

5 Drops Lavender Essential Oil

3 Tbsp Sweet Almond Oil

- Mix the dry ingredients and set aside
- Mix the oils together and add to the dry ingredients
- Place in container with a tight lid overnight
- Place an 1/8 cup of the salts in running water and mix well.

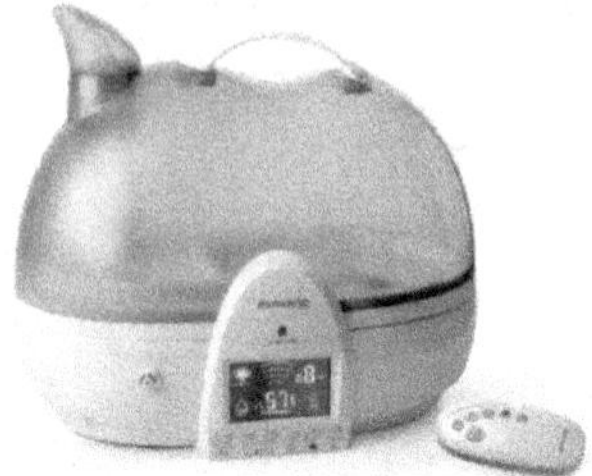

Sometimes it is best to have diffuser blends. These blends are placed either in a diffuser or a candle warmer. The release of the aroma of the blend will be inhaled as it travels through the air.

Newborn Immune Booster Blend

5 Drops Roman Chamomile Essential Oil

3 Drops Lavender Essential Oil

2 Drops Yarrow Essential Oil

1/4 cup Filtered Water

- Mix all ingredients well and place in diffuser
- Leave out the water and place 5 drops on a candle warmer

5-12 Year Immune Booster Blend

5 Drops Lavender Essential Oil

3 Drops Clary Sage Essential Oil

2 Drops Nutmeg Essential Oil

1/4 cup Filtered Water

- Mix all ingredients well and place in diffuser
- Leave out the water and place 5 drops on a candle warmer.

Chapter 4 - Dry Skin

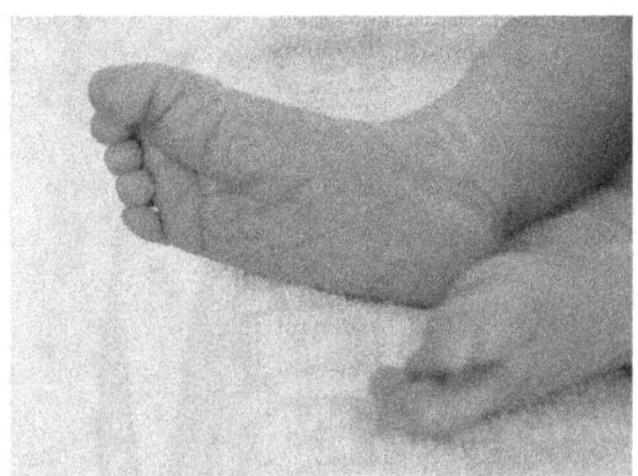

The dry patches, redness, and irritation that comes along with dry skin can be frustrating to us, but can you imagine how bad it can be to your child, especially when you tell them *not* to scratch the rash? Rashes can be due to poison ivy or some allergic reaction to something either ingested or that touched the skin. Rashes can be as simple as a small reddish patch on the skin to more severe cases like eczema or psoriasis. The good news they are treatable and avoidable if they are allergic reactions. To find out if your child has any allergies, you can take them to their pediatrician and ask for an allergen test.

Rashes can also be caused by stress and nervousness. If you child gets anxious when they have to speak in from of a class or large group of people or even be introduced to new people, they can develop a anxiety related skin condition. There is always a reason for the rash, and often that reason is a simple one.

Bathing in lukewarm or cool water will help the skin retain moisture while hot water will dry it out. Think about it for a minute. When you boil water, the meat shrinks as does any vegetable you boil in it. The same concept applies to your skin. It will wrinkle and not have the same elastic quality it should, making it easy to get cuts and rashes.

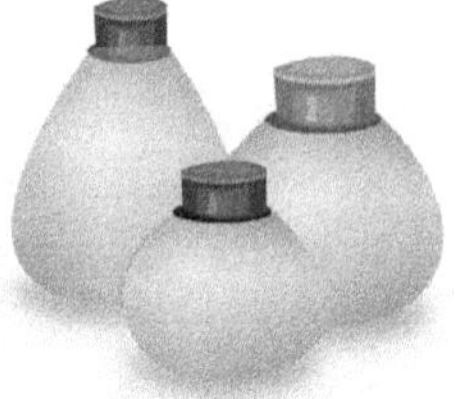

You can purchase the lotion base already made to save you the trouble. You can find it in hobby shops and online. You will also need a bottle to store the lotion. Here are a couple of lotion recipes you can use for your little one.

Newborn Rash Cream

2 ounces of lotion base

10 Drops Lavender Essential Oil

5 Drops Roman Chamomile Essential Oil

Mix all the ingredients together using a hand mixer and pour into the container. Place a small amount on the rash. If using on diaper rash, avoid the genital area.

12 Month to 5 Years Poison Ivy Cream

2 ounces of lotion base

10 Drops Palmarosa Essential Oil

5 Drops Roman Chamomile Essential Oil

5 Drops Tea Tree Essential Oil

Mix all the ingredients together using a hand mixer and pour into the container. Place a small amount on the rash. If using on diaper rash, avoid the genital area.

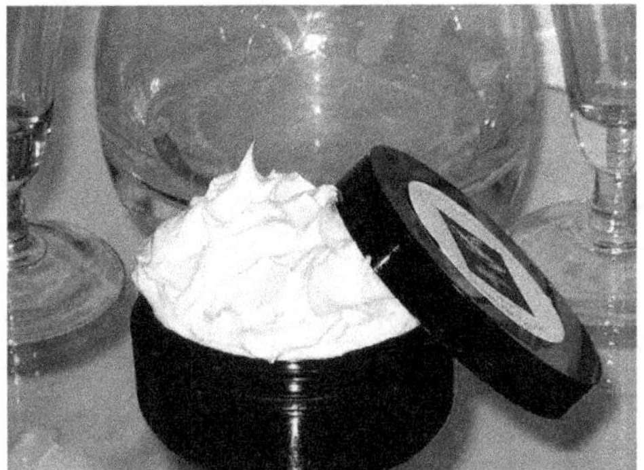

These are often found at stores in short, round containers and come in avocado, shea and other butters. Much like the lotion base, you can also find them online. You can also mix them together to increase effectiveness. You can make lotions for eczema or psoriasis, but body butters will last longer on the skin allowing the essential oils to stay on the area longer. You can also prevent the butter from rubbing off by having them wear a glove or wrapping the area with a bandage.

2 12 Months ema Psoriasis

1 Ounce Avocado Butter

1 Ounce Shea Butter

10 Drops Geranium Essential Oil

5 Drops Roman Chamomile Essential Oil

5 Drops Yarrow Essential Oil

- Mix the Butters and set aside
- Mix the essential oils and set aside
- Using a hand mixer, blend the essential oils into the butters
- Place the butter in an air-tight container

5-12 Years Eczema Psoriasis

1 Ounce Avocado Butter

1 Ounce Shea Butter

10 Drops Palmarosa Essential Oil

5 Drops Tea Tree Essential Oil

5 Drops Lavender Essential Oil

5 Drops Roman Chamomile Essential Oil

- Mix the Butters and set aside
- Mix the essential oils and set aside
- Using a hand mixer, blend the essential oils into the butters
- Place the butter in an air-tight container

All-Purpose Lotion

These two lotions can be used on an everyday basis for those days the skin looks a little ashy or for out of the bath.

Newborn

2 Ounces Lotion Base
15 Drops Lavender Essential Oil

Mix them together well. You can use this before putting your newborn to bed to help them sleep.

2–12 Months

2 Ounces Lotion Base
5 Drops Tangerine/Mandarin Essential Oil
5 Drops Geranium Essential Oil
5 Drops Roman Chamomile Essential Oil

Chapter 5 Homework and Concentration

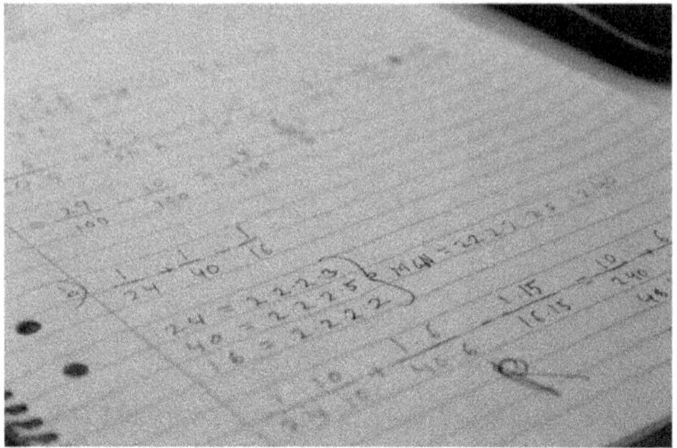

The hardest thing to do sometimes is getting your children to sit long enough to do their homework. They fidget, they squirm, and their focus tends to wane. Here are some things you can do to help them concentrate better.

1. Let them blow off some steam

Their fresh from having to sit for a few hours before they come home, and then there is the ride home, whether bus or car. Let them play for a bit before starting their homework. This lets them expend any extra energy, and they will fidget less. The best time for them to do their homework is normally after dinner.

2. Sit with them

Help them do their homework or just sit with them as they do it. You can read a book, write in a journal or anything else you can think of, but sitting with them as they do their homework will let them know you are there if they happen to get stuck.

□□No □istra□tions

Turn the Television off and confiscate their phone and other electronic devices. All these serve to distract them from getting their work done. If they need a calculator, by them a simple one or one suited to help them do the math they are currently practicing. If they want music, play jazz or classical. Soothing tones can help keep energy evened out and their mind on the task at hand.

These blends are focused on leveling out energy and toning down fidgeting. These are all diffuser blends for children 12 months to 12 Years.

Con□entration □□en□I

5 Drops Lavender Essential Oil
5 Drops Tangerine/Mandarin Essential Oil

Con□entration □□en□II

5 Drops Roman Chamomile Essential Oil
5 Drops Tangerine/Mandarin Essential Oil

They act out, come home with endless notes on behavior and can't seem to sit still for anything, and you have tried everything short of tying them to a chair. You're at the end of your rope, and so you take your child to the doctor, and after a battery of testing, they tell you your child has either ADD or ADHD. It's not the end of the world. You now know the problem. Here are some things you can do help them.

1□Re□□e s□□ars an□arti□i□ia□a□□itives in the □iet

This may seem like an insurmountable task, but switching to an all natural diet will help immensely. Don't know how to start? Feingold.org can help with that. Feingold is a doctor that was able to prove many learning disabilities stem from a diet laden with artificial preservatives, flavors, and colors. The website can walk you through the steps on living a life free of those.

2□□ive them a □itt□e □a□□eine□

Hear me out. When you give caffeine to a hyper child, they slow down and calm down. I know it sounds incredulous, but it's true. Caffeine acts like a depressant in the systems of those who suffer from ADD and ADHD.

Pe□□ermint □Mentha Pi□erita□

I am introducing this essential oil here because it does help with concentration and nervous tension. I have used several times when I have needed to stay on task.
The following blends are for ages 5 years and up.

ADD Blend I

5 Drops Peppermint Essential Oil
5 Drops Lavender Essential Oil

Blend well and either put five drops on a candle warmer or follow the directions for a diffuser.

ADD Blend II

3 Drops Peppermint Essential Oil
2 Drops Geranium Essential Oil
5 Drops Tangerine/Mandarin Essential Oil

Chapter Bedtime and Nervousness

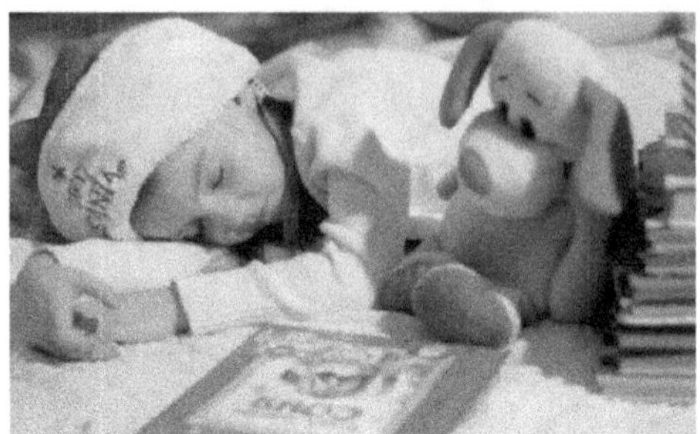

All of us who are parents know one simple truth about children. It's a battle to get them to go to bed. They don't want to miss anything and will *do* anything to stay up "Just a little bit longer". From asking for one more story to wanting to watch TV with you, there is no end to the negotiation at bedtime. Here are a couple of recipes you can use to help them drift off to sleep.

Hyperactivity Blend I

5 drops Chamomile Essential Oil
5 Drops Geranium Essential Oil
In a diffuser or candle warmer.

Hyperactivity Blend II

5 Drops Tangerine/Mandarin Essential Oil
5 Drops Chamomile Essential Oil

Whether it's the night before a big test or right before a recital or game, kids are a bundle of nerves and nervous energy. Here are a couple of recipes to help them calm down before those events.

Nervous Blend I

2 Drops Clary Sage Essential Oil

3 Drops Pepperminy Essential Oil

5 Drops Tangerine/Mandarin Essential Oil

Nervous Blend II

3 Drops Lavender Essential Oil

3 Drops Tangerine Essential Oil

2 Drops Geranium Essential Oil

2 Drops Clary Sage Essential Oil

Sleep Aid I

5 Drops Yarrow Essential Oil

3 Drops Chamomile Essential Oil

2 Drops Tangerine/Mandarin Essential Oil

Sleep Aid II

3 Drops Geranium Essential Oil

3 Drops Peppermint Essential Oil

4 Drops Yarrow Essential Oil

Cha□ter □□ath □ime

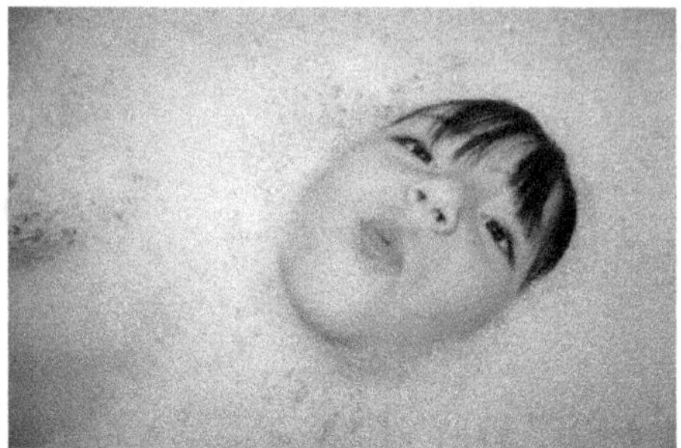

Kids get dirty. We can dress them up and they seem to attract dirt in a matter of seconds. Finding the right products to keep them clean without tons of chemicals is tricky. You can buy plain shampoo base from health retailers online.

Shampoo for Oily hair 5 Years+

4 Ounces Shampoo base

10 Drops Geranium Essential Oil

10 Drops Tangerine/Mandarin Essential Oil

Mix well and use as normal.

Shampoo 2-12 Months Oily Hair

2 Ounces Shampoo base

10 Drops Geranium Oil

5 Drops Lavender Essential Oil

Mix well and use as normal.

Dry Shampoo 2-12 mos

2 Ounces Shampoo base
10 Drops Chamomile Essential Oil
5 Drops Lavender Essential Oil

□i□e

The ban of every parent of school age children, lice are insidious. They get everywhere if not treated.

Lice Shampoo I 5 years+

4 Ounces Shampoo base
10 Drops Palmarosa Essential Oil
10 Drops Tea Tree Essential Oil
5 Drops Clary Sage Essential Oil

Lice Shampoo II 5 years+

4 Ounces Shampoo base
10 Drops Lavender Essential Oil
10 Drops Tangerine/Mandarin Essential Oil
5 Drops Tea Tree Oil Essential Oil

Body Soap for newborns

4 Ounces Goat's Milk Melt and Pour Soap
15 Drops Lavender Essential Oil
- Melt the soap in a double boiler
- Pour the soap in a mold
- Add the essential oil in when the soap is warm and you can still stir it

Soap for Boys 5+

4 Ounces Olive Oil Melt and Pour Soap

10 Drops Tangerine/Mandarin Essential Oil

10 Drops Palmarosa Essential Oil

5 Drops Clary Sage Essential Oil

Girls' Soap ages 5 and up Dry Skin

4 Ounces Goat's Milk Melt and Pour Soap

10 Drops Lavender Essential Oil

10 Drops Peppermint Essential Oil

5 Drops Palmarosa Essential Oil

• Mix the essential oils before you add them to the soap.

Girls' Soap ages 5 and up Oily Skin

4 Ounces Goat's Milk Melt and pour Soap

10 Drops Tangerine/Mandarin Essential Oil

10 Drops Geranium Essential Oil

5 Drops Palmarosa Essential Oil

• Mix the essential oils before you add them to the soap.

Facial Care

As they get older, kids need a different soap to cleanse their faces. Here are a few recipes you can use. All of these are for children ages 5 and up.

Recipe I (for pimples)

4 Ounces Olive Oil Melt and Pour

5 Drops Eucalyptus Essential Oil

10 Drops Palmarosa Essential oil

5 Drops Tea Tree Essential Oil

5 Drops Lavender Essential Oil

Recipe II (Oily Skin)

4 Ounces Goat's Milk Melt and Pour Soap

10 Drops Tangerine/Mandarin Essential Oil

10 Drops Geranium Essential Oil

5 Drops Clary Sage Essential Oil

Recipe III (Dry Skin)

4 Ounces Goat's Milk Melt and Pour Soap

10 Drops Lavender Essential Oil

10 Drops Chamomile Essential Oil

5 Drops Yarrow Essential Oil

Cha□ter □□i□s an□□ri□□s

Here is a list of quick things you can do when you don't have all of the ingredients to make the recipes.

1. You can add 3 drops to every tablespoon of shampoo to help treat lice.

2. You can add 3 drops of Lavender essential oils to every tablespoon of liquid soap to sooth your infant's nerves before bed. This will help them sleep.

3. To help speed healing in cases of sunburn, add 3 drops of Lavender to each tablespoon of Aloe gel.

4. Three drops of Eucalyptus on your child's night light before plugging it in will help them breathe better when they have a cold.

It doesn't stop there

You can find forums online to help further your knowledge of essential oils and aromatherapy. You can find new recipes, get advice, and even suggest some of your own. There is no end to the learning.

Conclusion

I hope the information in this book has helped get you started in your new and rewarding facet of natural health. There are a myriads of books and sites you can use to continue your education. Until next time, stay well.

www.ingramcontent.com/pod-product-compliance
Lightning Source LLC
Chambersburg PA
CBHW070750260726
48660CB00007B/3053

PROSENCE
QUALITY OVER QUANTITY

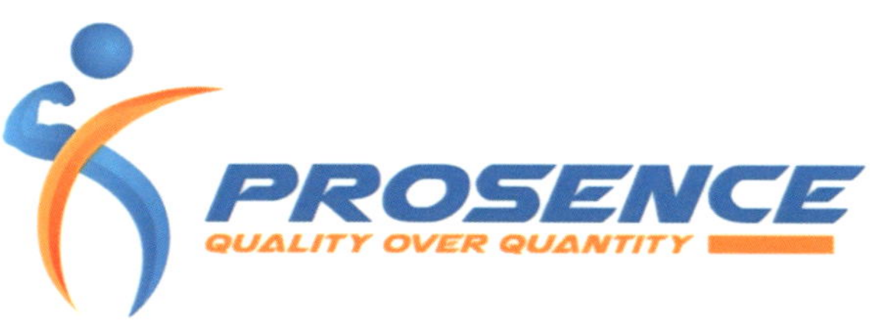

HIIT

What It Is and Why It Works

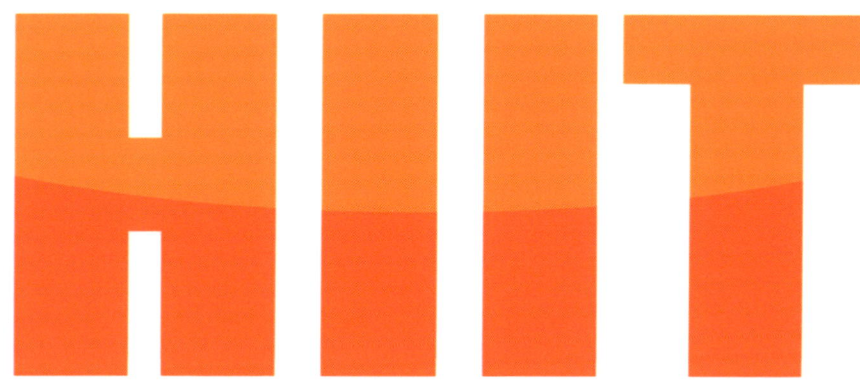

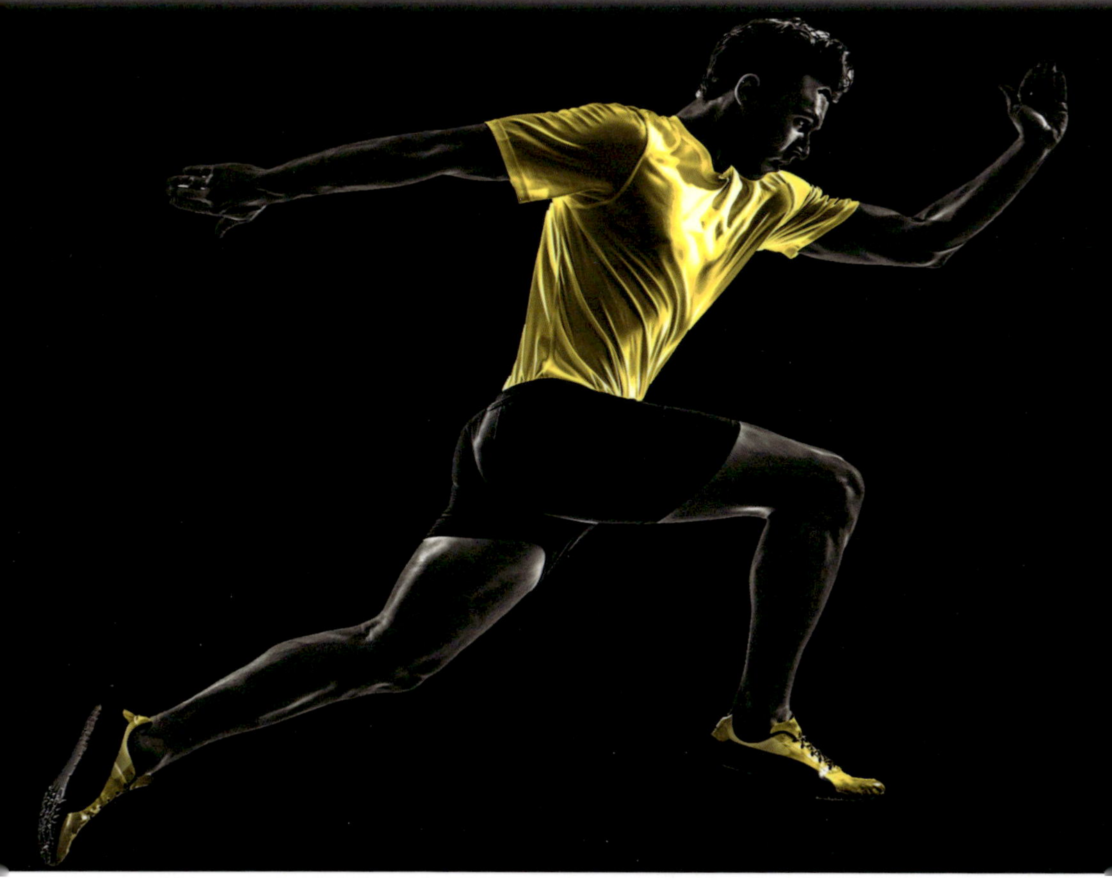